EFFORTLESS DIET

I0425531

The Complete Guide to Lose Weight for Beginners, Gain Energy & Stay Healthy. Intermittent Fasting and Ketogenic diet

HAILEY.T

ISBN: 9781091853041

Table of Contents

Preface

Weight loss is a journey, not just a weekend trip. That being said, it is going to take some time to actually achieve your goals. You likely won't find it to be an easy, casual journey either. You are going to run into some bumps and slipups that might make it hard to recover. There are going to be moments when you ask if it is worth it all in the end and other times where you question why you are even doing what you are. It is not going to be an easy or quick thing. If it were, you would have done it by now.

Keep in mind that there is no one way for weight loss solutions. Everybody's approach, ability and outcome are different but the motivation is common to achieving a healthy body and mind. People tend to ignore the fact that there is more to weight loss than just calorie count and exercises. Your mindset, diet, exercise and lifestyle habits play important roles as well, in fact very subtly but powerfully! All these aspects should be synergized to work together in order to achieve effective results maximally.

Each chapter here will help you look at the process of losing weight in a very practical and inspiring way. Losing weight is undeniably not an easy task but always remember that challenges can be surmounted with baby steps taken within your comfort level, and then slowly but surely moving yourself up. Allow yourself to be surprised by what you can do to your own body. It's in your DNA to want to outdo yourself! So why not do it?

This book is dedicated to all women who want to find the path to losing weight. Here, we present to you guaranteed and assuring ways to bring your weight down in the most do-able manner that fits your lifestyle and in your comfort level. Something that you won't have to sacrifice so much that you don't even feel like starting the journey.

All of this is important to accept when beginning a weight-loss regimen. Accept the fact that there is no small fix for weight loss. There are pills you can take that help a bit, and other supplements that might help you lose some pounds. To really change your life and finally become the person you have always wanted to be, however, it is going to take some time. Weight loss is a process that requires patience, acceptance, and dedication. Though it might be tough at first, it does get easier. Achieving your goals is ALWAYS worth it in the end.

All you have to keep in mind is that patience, persistence and consistency are key. You will want to stop, you will want to quit, you will want to eat more and you will want to give up but YOU HAVE THE WILLPOWER TO RESIST AND START AFRESH EVERYTIME!

Let's start this journey together and reach the finishing line together

Weight loss can be one of the most annoying things you may want to accomplish in your life, but it is worth it. Exercise, eating a specific way, having to govern yourself in certain situations and be regimented is not easy. If weight loss was always easy none of us would have to do it. The great news is that weight loss can be a goal you set and achieve.

Maintaining a nice weight for your height and size is so possible, you can start right now. You basically have started by reading this book.

This book was written to help you identify what you already know to be true for weight loss but have maybe forgotten. For some you, it will be new information. What it takes to lose weight is sometimes so simple we do not think it possible. This book is here to guide you back to where your body wants to be for health, feeling good, and doing more and more in this world.

Your Own Story-Intelligent Women=Intelligent Diet=Effortless Get In Shape

Chapter 1: Why did you fail to lose weight

There is a root issue for why someone can't lose weight. Food for some people becomes a comfort that not everyone is ready to let go of. Whether someone hates eating veggies and only eats junk, or if someone binges healthy food, there is a reason why we all have our certain eating habits. By digging deep into our past, present, and goals for the future, we can discover that the key to losing weight is not in a pill or program. It is all in our head.

The only tool necessary to lose weight is your brain. You can find ways to work out without any gear or extra supplements. These certainly help make things easier, and many people find help from having different tools of motivation. The key—the most important tool of all—is a mindset that is ready to confront the issues and work through them in order to achieve weight-loss goals.

Having a clear goal as well as a plan of attack are the next two important tools needed to make sure that you are going to be able to lose the weight once and for all, as well as the tools needed to make sure the weight does not come back.

To begin, you first need to change the way you look at weight loss. To do that, you need to look at how you view failure.

Let me caution you, this is not always going to be easy. Staying focused, constantly thinking positively, savoring every victory, and forgetting the missteps is just part of the process necessary to reach that ultimate goal – losing weight and maintaining a lifelong healthy lifestyle.

Will you reach that day when all the world is rose-colored and you will never have to think about weight loss again? NO! This is my point. This book is not to solely help you reach your weight loss goals – there are hundreds of thousands of those books available. I want you to see your life differently. I want you to take on this program – not as a weight loss guide – but a change-of-life guide.

You now know that you will never fail, because you're NEVER going to give-up. RIGHT? Say the following aloud – several times a day, EVERY DAY: "I Will Never Give Up! I Will Look at All Setbacks as Just Another Failed Attempt, But Not a Failure. I Will See These Setbacks Simply as Challenges and Learning Experiences That Will Ultimately Lead Me to My Success!!"

Weight loss obsession-Over Thinking About Weight Loss

The mental toll of reaching your weight loss goal can also be the source of your stress. When the stress caused by over thinking about weight loss becomes too high, it may also cause your motivation to work out to dwindle.

Success in weight loss can be achieved if you are doing the exercises needed to be done without taking much of your time thinking about it and that's where the need for mindfulness arises. Mindfulness is the practice of becoming completely aware of the present instead of dwelling on the past or venturing into the future. It is a way of clearly seeing and paying attention to what is happening around you. While it cannot get rid of the pressure you experience, it can help you respond to it in a better and calmer manner. Mindfulness can help you recognize and stay away from unconscious physiological and emotional reactions to daily events. It can provide you with a scientific approach to cultivating insight, understanding, and clarity. When you practice mindfulness, you will be able to be completely present in your life and even improve its quality.

When it's time to work out for instance, you are only focused on that task instead of thinking the number of pounds you will lose after the activity. For very important thoughts, you need to have a piece of paper and write them down in a list. The less important thoughts on the other hand should be released. The idea is to get your focus back on the task at hand as soon as possible.

Wrong Mind

The way we think is a major part of how we lose weight. Our bodies do whatever we tell them to do, so if we are not thinking to do what we are supposed to everyday to be healthy, fit, and rested then we can get ourselves into trouble. It is important to just wipe your mind clean of what you think about weight loss and try to follow the simple rules in this book to get yourself to the target weight you desire to be happy.

It is important to be realistic that you want to be the healthiest version of yourself. This means coming to terms that you may want to look like a movie star or some other person, because you think they look good or have things you want, but you can have everything you want under your own terms. You have to be realistic about what your weight loss will look like. It is not about you trying to look like someone else. It is about you looking as good as you can in terms of healthy hair, good teeth, nice skin, muscle mass, and energy. This is what looks good. Looking good means being healthy. Health and energy is what we usually notice in beautiful people.

There is a misconception of the more you do the skinnier you will be or better looking you will be and this is false. Although everyone is very different sometimes when people do just enough they are healthier this way than if they try to do too much. Sometimes people do not lose weight, because they are doing too much. Exhausting yourself can cause a physical reaction that does not help you lose weight. The goal to a beautiful mind and body is one of balance between rest and activity, water and food. Food means a balance between healthy food and giving yourself the treats, sweets, and fattening foods in moderation so that you do not feel denied things you want to eat. Portion is key.

Your emotions and others comments can play tricks on yours to throw you out if balance. Work can throw you off balance. It is important to keep your mind focused on life balance to attain and maintain a healthy weight.

Wrong Method-Why Most Diets Fail

Most diet plans are not based on good science. In many cases they are misleading as is evidenced by their short-term effect with secondary weight gain. In fact, most diets which work for rapid weight loss also create a disastrous metabolism effect so that weight gain automatically returns with a vengeance! Just remember that the real value of a diet has nothing to do with short term weight loss. If short-term weight loss were your primary goal, then you could achieve it through starvation, stimulant prescriptions, drug use, jaw wiring, etc., all of which have harmful, long-term side effects on health and jeopardize the body's ability to sustain weight loss. On the other hand, weight loss programs that are healthy and result in sustained weight loss require complete dietary and lifestyle changes. To be successful, the participant has to closely monitor everything that goes into his or her mouth. They must closely follow the principals we have outlined in this book including, diet, exercise, stress management, and sleep. In our society it is very difficult to follow such a regimen. A very small proportion of the food that is normally purchased at the grocery store or at most restaurants is adequate, most of it is laden with undesirable, fat causing ingredients. Daily and sustained exercise programs are time and energy consuming. Life is full of various stressors that are sometimes very difficult to avoid and many of us are frequently deprived of an optimal amount of sleep for various reasons.

The real value of a diet plan should have nothing to do with short-term weight loss. The truth is, most "lose weight quick" diets will help you drop a few pounds relatively fast. These rapid weight-loss schemes wreak havoc on your metabolism—and that's a *guaranteed* setup for weight to return with a vengeance! There's very little chance you'll be able to keep the weight off, which makes all your hard work virtually *worthless*!

Finding The "WHY" In Your Diet

Let's get to the "WHY" factor – which, in my opinion, is the single most important element necessary to succeed in anything in life that requires motivation, endurance, perseverance, and aspiration. And why I believe finding the true underlying reason, why you want to lose weight or change your lifestyle is the key to your success, as it was mine.

When considering your "WHY", I want you to focus on YOUR reasons for wanting to lose weight. What is important to you? Losing weight, adopting healthy eating habits, changing your lifestyle – all MUST be done for YOU!

Your reasoning may be because you are finally tired of looking the way you do, or your health requires it, or you are afraid of what your loss may do to your family. All of these reasons are YOUR reasons. They are important to YOU.

You will not find success because your spouse thinks you should lose 50 pounds, or your parents are telling you that you need to lose weight. While outside influences can certainly push us toward finding our "WHY", they cannot be THE "WHY". You are searching for that "WHY" factor that has ultimately brought you to a point of desperation.

Once you have discovered your "WHY", you will be tapping into that "WHY" daily; using that "WHY" to help you alter your bad lifestyle choices and morph them into good - permanent - lifestyle choices.

Making a few healthy changes and educating yourself will keep you focused as you make more changes, (and always at a pace in which you are comfortable), but more so, you will find that you want to make them, which ultimately aids your progress and keeps you on a positive track.

So, to get started, I would like you to find a quiet place, where you can close your eyes and just relax for several minutes. Remember this is about you, not anyone else. Remind yourself, you are a good person and you deserve this time to focus on you.

Wrong target-failure due to lack of motivation

Don't choose to focus on positive or negative fantasies about your future self. Instead, focus on both. Doublethink everything, looking for the bad side as well as the good.

Do train yourself to realize that, at some point, your willpower is going to disappear. Instead of wallowing in misery, tell people what your goals are and ask for support to lower the chance of you failing.

Don't stick to picking a goal; pick all of its sub goals as well. The goal is what you want to achieve, the sub goals are how you are going to achieve it.

Look for the right role model. If you are scared of failing, then look for a role model who has failed. It is their story that will inspire you to succeed

Don't ever beat yourself up if you eat something that's not allowed. The power of regret is far more powerful if you use it before you do something or if you fail to do something than it is if you wait until afterwards

The most important thing is to realize that no motivational technique on earth is a magic pill. They can't make you lose weight, only you can do that and, if you don't really want to then you won't. If you do, then you have taken the first step and these motivational techniques will help you to succeed.

The most important mind hack is the utmost support and care from your family and friends. Make sure you inform all your loved ones about your weight loss goals right from the beginning so that they are also committed to reminding you and encouraging you along the way. Words of encouragement from your family can be a great kick start to your journey. It can help you deal with the challenges that come with the weight loss process, and at any point, pull you up to regain your confidence and the will to do better.

Remember their positive messages and gestures and try to update them on your journey as well. Make sure that you avoid those family or friends who are negative towards your weight loss experience. Have the wisdom to discard their unhelpful or insensitive remarks. Also, avoid social activities that involve dining out at new cafes or restaurants or clubbing as this will inevitably provide you with lots of unnecessary temptations and regain the weight that you have lost. As much as you want to socialize, be smart to say 'no' to unhealthy food or friends if you love yourself more.

How you can succeed

Now, the sixty-four-million-dollar question, given all we have gone over so far, how can you succeed in a sustainable weight loss program? We know for sure that if you strictly adhere to the diet, exercise, stress reduction, and sleep hygiene principles we discussed earlier you will definitely be successful. Unfortunately, strictly adhering to all of these guidelines is difficult at best and nearly impossible for many of us at worst. Your next logical question may be, "Ok, so why do you mention all of these guidelines if most of us won't strictly adhere to them?" You must at least be aware of these principles and follow them to some extent in order to be successful. Do not be deceived, the more closely you follow these guidelines, the more successful you will be. Since most of us falter, we need some further assistance.

Why Your Body is Not Meant to Diet, And Why It's Not Your Fault

As women, our bodies are not meant to diet, or even worse, lose weight. It truly is harder for women to lose weight, and it makes total sense if you stop to think about it. Everything about our genetic make-up stems from way back in history from our time as hunters and gatherers.

Since the early stages of time, our ancestors have had to fight to survive. They didn't have ready-made foods and they definitely didn't have delivery! The men had to hunt and we women had to nurse and bear children.

In order to successfully survive, men needed to be as fast and as lean as possible in order to keep up with their animal counterparts. And in order to do that, their fat storages needed to be low. A man's DNA is meant to be a lean hunter and it almost goes against a man's DNA to store a lot of fat.

Lucky them!

Men, by nature, have more fat burning enzymes than women!

Us women on the other hand, now that's a whole different story. We have a very different DNA make-up, don't we? Our DNA was specifically designed for survival. We are built to survive times of famine and scarcity. It's like we were made to accumulate fat and to never lose those accumulations no matter how hard we try!

Well it's not "like" we are built this way, it is a FACT that we are built to bear children, produce milk, and to care for the children in times of scarcity and famine. Our entire genetic makeup is built around survival in harsh times and in times where food may not be sufficient. Our genetic makeup is built for survival, not to "look good" by today's standards. Losing weight goes against everything that makes us who we are!

Women have it a bit tougher than men. And this is the real reason why most diets don't work!

To take it a step further, when we diet, what we are really doing is sending a signal to our bodies that there is famine, and our bodies should hold on for dear life to preserve whatever fat it has left! Our fat burning enzymes slow down and even decrease in size. Sometimes up to 40%! This is the real reason why most diet plans will ultimately fail.

Know Your Body

Everybody is different from one another. And so are the ways our bodies react to certain changes as well. A weight loss journey for every person is different because our metabolic rates are individually personalized. Metabolic rate and genetics play a great role in losing weight. Some people find it easier to maintain their weight through a combination of exercise and proper nutrition but others may struggle to do so. Here are some things that you need to know about your body: People who are larger in size or have more muscle mass burn more calories even when they are resting. Males of the same weight and age as females, generally have more muscle mass and less body fat than females, thus burn more calories.

1. As you age, your muscle mass decreases. This process is termed as sarcopenia. You therefore burn calories slower than your younger counterparts.

2. Your genes are also a great definer. More than 400 genes have been linked by researchers to metabolism, cravings and fats distribution in the body. This means that some people may have lesser

cravings or they may have a faster metabolism. While others can have a natural weight distribution on certain body parts.

So, it is highly important that you understand your body and know what suits you. You can even visit a nutritionist if you cannot understand this by yourself. Learn your body right to get the right results!

How to Achieve Weight Loss Without Fail?

Weight loss can be a very goal oriented challenge and a good reason could be due to the foods you love too much to give up. If you are struggling with weight loss, you still have time to rectify the situation and get yourself in to a desired shape. Losing weight can be your ultimate key to better health and feeling good about yourself. You can cut down the risks of diabetes, heart attack, stroke, kidney failure and so many more health issues by taking the necessary steps to cut back on the extra fat that you may be carrying. You have a reason to live for yourself and your family by making a change today.

Things happen in life that can make for sudden changes in your lifestyle and body. Weight gain could be due to stress, eating disorders or even comfort to name some. Honestly, you can combat it all and free yourself to a better you. Changing the way, you eat and move can be very successful to achieve your goal. Weight loss can be achieved by anyone. It takes time and effort to achieve your goals. If you are one of the people who have said you have tried everything yet you see no results, the truth is you are not being as consistent as you should.

Having a cheat day in the middle or end of the week can break your efforts greatly because eating something you miss can lure you right back into the position you first started from. Sometimes it's hard to give up on the foods you love but you have to reason with yourself and break the habit. Who's the boss? You or the food?

Do you love fast food? If so, the fat and salt content can be very damaging to your health especially if you eat it every day. Weight gain will come without a doubt if you consume too much.

If you don't know what foods to consume to help you lose weight, the following ideas can help you be off to a great start on your weight loss journey. Remember that when you start this journey, be very serious and consistent about it because making the wrong decisions by trying to cheat yourself will either leave you in the same situation or add more weight to what you already have.

Chapter 2: An Inspirational Story

Get fit in a lazy and smart way-you deserve it

Take a deep breath and exhale through your nose slowly. Repeat this several times, and each time, concentrate on relaxing your neck, chest, arms, back, abdomen, legs, feet, and your mind. Continue focusing until you are relaxed.

While keeping, your eyes closed, I want you to focus on what has brought you here. At this point, it will most likely cause you to think of every negative thought that has been a part of your weight issues. This is good – as long as you are thinking of these negatives for what they are – the stumbling blocks; the hurdles; the failed attempts – all the things that have brought you here. Think hard about this and do not rush your answer.

What are your motivators? Are you feeling physically limited, are you having breathing problems, are you diabetic, or fear becoming diabetic, are you disgusted by your appearance once and for all, is your weight putting your family at risk, is your weight jeopardizing your job?

Once you have faced all of the reasons why you want to lose weight, I want you to focus on all of them – each one separately, and jointly. Ultimately, what does it all boil down to? What is the sole reason you NEED to lose weight? THIS IS YOUR "WHY"! FOCUS ON THIS!! Keep thinking about that "WHY". Embed it in your mind. Ingrain it in your memory bank. Your "WHY" will become your life!

Write that answer down under Step 1 – MY WHY - "Why do I want to lose weight or get into better shape?" Read it back to yourself – again and again. Quantify your answer. Is this truly your reason for making a lifestyle change?

Close your eyes again and take a couple deeper breaths and relax. Concentrate once again on your "WHY", and let's dig deeper into that "WHY". Why is your "WHY" important to you? This is important. Why is this "WHY" the root that will keep you focused on wanting a healthier lifestyle? Concentrate on this, and remember this about yourself.

Again, I stress – YOU CANNOT DO THIS FOR ANYONE ELSE BUT YOU! Do not take what I just said wrong. Again, your "WHY" might be because you want to look better for someone else and that is ok, if that is important to YOU.

Write down the reason this is important to you under "Why is that important to me"? Read it back to yourself. Now return to the first question, reread your answer, and then reread the reason your "WHY" is important to you. Read them aloud. Do you hear yourself? Are you quantifying these responses? Does the "WHY" sound like the REAL reason you want to change your lifestyle? Is this reason really important to you?

If you are struggling with the first two steps, perhaps we need to dig a bit deeper. Again, take another deep breath and relax. This time, when you think about the "WHY" and the reason the "WHY" is important to you? When you do this, dig really deep into your emotions and your past. What kind of pain has been overweight or out of shape caused you?

Be like a boss-confident Mastered

Keeping things in is never good. In fact, it can feel pretty awful. Those that are overweight might find themselves feeling embarrassed about their weight. Maybe they end up making excuses for themselves when they eat certain foods, verbalizing these reasons to others around them as a form of validation. "Oh, I'll just start my diet tomorrow," you might hear someone say as they sneak a few extra cupcakes from the dessert table. This kind of discussion can be counterintuitive. Instead, try talking about the issues and struggles you have rather than about the way you're going to make up for your problems later. You might find that you end up getting some great advice from a person that's going through a similar struggle.

It's important to be a good listener as well. Sometimes, people aren't looking for answers or advice when they're complaining about their issues. It's nice to just have someone to vent to every once in a while. By creating a discussion, you can more easily tackle the issues that are causing problems in your weight-loss journey.

Avoid telling people about your goal before you get on track, however. Talking about your feelings, emotions, and struggles is always a good thing. Sometimes it just takes saying a thing out loud for it to feel real. However, many people set themselves up for failure by sharing their goals too early. Those that post on social media about how they're going to lose weight are actually less likely to follow through with their goals. Stay silent with the majority in the beginning of your journey, confiding in just those you know you can rely on and trust.

Spreading positive Thoughts-Positive Affirmations

An affirmation is a type of positive reinforcement that helps in combating negative thoughts. If you're like most of us, you already know negative affirmations work. We have all heard them – either from others or from ourselves. Many, many of us were bullied as children, received negative comments from teachers or parents or friends, and those negative thoughts played like a rerun in our minds – for many years.

And, unfortunately, the negative affirmations worked to keep us believing these negative comments. Why, because we tend to repeat the negative affirmations to ourselves over and over and over again. And, we repeat the negative affirmations even more so than we do positive affirmations. Negative affirmations just seem to be more prevalent in our lives. Why? Because we all tend to be our own worst critics, in which we affirm everything that is not 'perfect' about ourselves.

But, the more we think about them, the more we repeat them, the more we allow ourselves to believe them. I mean, let's face reality - all we have to do is look in the mirror to receive confirmation that these affirmations are 'real'. Over a period of time, those negative affirmations will become our standard thinking pattern.

Those negative beliefs have become so deeply engrained in our subconscious minds that we have come to believe them, and no positive affirmation reverses that self-image.

Constructive affirmations or constructive self-talk not only serve to your advantage but also to other individuals with whom you have any communication. Affirmation is the reversal of beliefs rooted in negative, messy, and cruel events from our past to a more positive mindset. The success achieved from committing to positive affirmations will change your "I can't do it" attitude to "I can do anything". And that, my friends, will be the secret to your success.

If you are of the belief, as many are, that constructive affirmations have its influence only on the intuitive personality, I offer an opportunity to present evidence to the contrary.

Beside muscle quality, positive affirmations also have a direct influence on your vitality level. An upbeat individual is typically a depiction of the consequences related to a positive personality programming.

So, the bottom line is this - unless we remove the negative affirmations and replace them with strong, positive affirmations, confirming our self-worth and the belief that we can achieve anything - we will forever be stuck in our current life. There will never be a resolve to our weight problems. Positive affirmations are as important to your success as your "WHY"!

Positivity is your fuel throughout this process to pump you up to your optimal stage before and during your entire weight loss journey.

First and foremost, you need to create positive affirmations. Positive affirmations are considered to be the language of the brain because once the brain picks on them it becomes a constant mantra of the mind. And just like language, it comes naturally to us whenever we feel low or we feel like giving up on ourselves. Affirmations help you send positive messages to your unconscious mind so that you start to reiterate these positive thoughts to yourself when in need.

Practicing affirmations is an important mindset strategy in weight loss. Instead of telling yourself you're "no good" because you didn't follow through with a small goal, you should give yourself an affirmation such as "I am capable of continuing" to remind yourself of how powerful you really are. Below is a list of positive affirmations you should use in order to combat negative thoughts and improve overall encouragement:

- I can do this. I am capable of losing weight and I have the ability to reach my goals.
- I am exercising every day and eating healthy as often as possible. I am actually doing what I should be doing in order to achieve my goals.
- If I can start my journey, I can finish it.
- I do not need processed foods to feel happy. I can feel the same joy from cooking a healthy meal.
- I have exercised before and can do it again. It is hard to start, but I know that once I do, I have what it takes to finish my exercise routine.

- I am healing myself. I have been through challenging times and deserve to feel happy.
- I am loved and am full of love.
- I am losing weight to be healthy.
- I am beautiful no matter what size. Skipping one day at the gym does not mean that I am not beautiful.
- I am eating healthy food full of nourishment. I can feel the positive change in my body and I know that I only have more to look forward to.

Moving Forward

To the credit of my lifestyle change, I am now leaner, stronger, healthier, and happier than I have been in many years. I no longer feel 'disabled' by my disabilities. I have learned to use those disabilities as reasons to keep going. My battle to lose weight was not easy and will never stop, but I made it fun. And I know the next time something in my life causes me to lose my motivation and gain weight, I will be able to stop it before I gain all the weight back and I will again be able to find my WHY and start again. If you will follow the steps in this book to find your WHY and you can find the fun and excitement in learning new ways to live healthy as I did, I promise you that success will be yours as well.

This book, was written to assist those that want to lose weight, want to live healthier, want to live happier, but just haven't been able to find the key to success. I hope this book shows you the importance of knowing your "WHY", and why that "WHY" must supersede everything else in your life.

- Do this for your health!
- Do this for your happiness!
- Do this for your future!
- Do this for YOU!

If the information in this book provides you with that one component that has been missing in every previous failed attempt tried, I have served my purpose. I have the utmost respect for you, and I know you can do this! You just need to know that you can do!

Chapter 3: Set Goals

What can our minds do? Of all the successful people we have ever met or all their interviews we have read, they always emphasize how powerful our minds can be.

Our minds are extremely powerful weapons that are lying dormant most of the time. Imagine the innumerable benefits if you can gain access and program your brain to work the way that you want it so as to achieve your goals and dreams.

Goals and Consciously Keeping Track

It is important to have a certain body goal in mind. Without the goal, your weight loss process is just a futile effort which has no end result. If you keep certain goals or gain any inspiration from your favorite celebrity, you will be able to work towards them gradually.

Furthermore, keep weekly and daily goals. These goals will help you achieve your target in no time. It will also help you keep track of your success and failures. When you set the benchmark, you can channel your activities towards reaching the goals and this can help you to be clearer about how much effort you need to put in. Some of the daily or weekly goals can be about:

1.   The calories you will eat throughout the day (if you are into calorie count).

2. It can be your daily step counts (Get a step tracker watch! Affordable ones are available in online stores! Aim to achieve 7k-10k steps daily is good.)

3. Your weekly exercise schedule (3 times a week for 30 minutes at least? Or do you prefer 10 minutes daily? Monday evening, or Sunday morning preferred?)

4. Your weekly targeted exercise drills. (1 set of 15 minutes skipping; 1 set of 15 minutes Zumba dance; 1 set of 15 minutes' static exercise?)

5. Have a food planner. Plan out your meals in it, keep a calories count and what you would like to eat on your cheat days, apart from that you can note down helpful recipes as well.

You cannot achieve a healthy lifestyle overnight. This needs time, patience and a considerable amount of physical and mental energy. Stay strong and motivated with yourself. Short-term goals help to keep you on track and see the light at the end of the tunnel.

Now, go get a nice journal book just for this weight loss journey! Start writing down your positive affirmations, meditation schedule, initial measurements and the daily or weekly goals that you want to achieve. Review them constantly, make amendments if need be.

Staying On Track

The moment you start your weight loss journey; it is very important to keep track of your progress. This can sometimes be frustrating when you are not getting desired results but this should not discourage you.

In order to keep track, you should maintain a journal or a diary that records your initial measurements consisting of your weight early in the morning, waist and hip inches. Measurements are important because they help us to objectively analyze our bodily changes. By maintaining this journal, you can keep adding entries on a daily or weekly basis according to what suits you best. So, once you complete a month or more, you can always go back to these entries and check the patterns and progress based on what you have done.

Looking Inward

Sometimes, our weight-loss goals are all about just making sure that we look good in a bikini. Though we want our outsides to look good, we have to make sure the insides are looking even better. This does not mean your bones and blood, but your heart and mind. Is your brain ready to go through such a journey? Is your heart really in it in the end?

If you want to make sure you look good, you can't expect to do so while completely disregarding the inner workings of all the other systems in your body. This journey should be a healthy one, and that does not mean just looking the part. Crash dieting, binging and purging, and using extreme weight-loss supplements are all just attempts at fixing something that weight loss will not cure.

What's more important than just making sure you can fit into the right-sized outfit for an upcoming wedding is making sure that your mental state is strong enough to handle it if you don't end up fitting. The first step in doing this is making sure that you look at the root issue rather than looking at what you see in the mirror.

Finding a New Goal

What's your goal for losing weight? Is it to fit into a dress? Is it so you can get a new boyfriend/girlfriend? Is it so you have a flat stomach or so your face is not as round? If your goal for losing weight is just to look good, you should find a new goal. That is the reason many people want to lose weight in the first place. They just want to be "hot" or "sexy," with a fit body that attracts other people, or at least gets positive attention from those around them. It is not uncommon to have vanity goals when it comes to losing weight. It is also not uncommon for people to give up on their weight-loss goals.

Looking good should just be an added bonus for losing weight. If you don't find a substantial and deeply-rooted goal for losing weight, you won't be as likely to keep up with your hopes. Instead of losing weight just to be hot, you have to find a reason that is more important.

Lose weight because you want to have a healthy heart. Having a healthy heart means that you will live longer, which means you'll get to spend more time with your friends and family. When you create a goal that has more meaning, you will be able to stick to that goal more easily than if you just want to be able to slip into some skinny jeans.

Create smaller goals that are important as well. Lose the weight because you want to be able to walk up a flight of stairs without having to catch your breath. Lose weight because you want to make it easier to move when it comes time to switch apartments. Lose weight because you will have the assurance that you can outrun anyone in case of some sort of zombie apocalypse.

35

Just remember that looking the best out of everyone at your high school reunion will just be the added bonus to losing weight, not the overall goal. That way, you will be able to stick to your weight-loss regimen if you do hit a certain body weight.

It is also important to understand your current value and beauty. You are not ugly, unattractive, or undesirable at any weight. That beautiful person exists inside of you, and it will show through no matter what size you are. You just have to recognize that wonderful person and treat them well, not shame them for not looking "sexy" enough.

When creating a goal, you have to look at the overall benefits that will come along with achieving certain milestones. By doing this, you will be able to fulfill your goals better because you have a clear map of what benefits you will be reaping.

There are so many benefits to losing weight besides just the way you might look. Losing weight could help someone manage with their anxiety and depression. Working out releases endorphins, and certain junk food has been linked to producing depressive feelings.

Being more in shape allows someone to do things that someone out of shape, can't. You can go for walks with friends and not have to worry about what games you might play that could involve physical activity.

Being an overweight teenager and young adult is challenging because, at that age, there is so much pressure to look good. However, being overweight and in your forties or older is so much worse, and not even for beauty reasons. As our bodies age, no matter how healthy they are, certain things just don't work the way they used to. Our backs, knees, and hips start to not work as well as they used to and being overweight just puts more pressure on all these parts of our bodies. The older you get, the harder being overweight is on your body. It is also harder to lose weight the older you get. Losing the weight now, no matter what age, is always a better option than waiting and losing the weight later.

How Is Weight Weighing You Down?

It is common knowledge that being overweight doesn't only come with physical health issues, it is almost always accompanied by many other issues *i.e.* social anxiety, lack of confidence, self-consciousness and low self-esteem. Weight is diminishing your physical and mental energy thus killing your potential. You are capable of great things! Your mind is a fast running machine but to keep up with its pace, you need to have a healthy fit body to carry you through. Don't let all the extra pounds weigh you down!

There is no secret that being overweight has innumerable disadvantages. When you're in one phase for a very long period, you tend to overlook the negative side and continue ignoring the problem. This results in finding comfort in the current situation which further results in a lack of motivation to eradicate that problem. This section is dedicated to giving you a reality check and bringing your attention to the ways weight gain is interfering with your life and weighing you down.

Weight is a big contributor to your mental well-being as well. If you're overweight or underweight, you can go into depression or take on bad eating habits of either starving yourself or overeating in order to get your ideal weight. The issues that overweight people often face are having self-loathing thoughts, negative thinking process and low self-esteem issues, to name a few.

What a waste if your body is disrupting the process of you achieving more than what you are capable of. What if I'm telling you that there are proven methods that you can gain control and execute to improve your weight and your overall life? Do you want to make it happen?

Small Wins and Losses

Having an overall goal is important, but make sure to set small goals in between. For example, maybe your overall goal is to lose fifty pounds in a year. A small goal, then, would be to lose five pounds. Instead of waiting to celebrate until you lose the big fifty, have five-or ten-pound milestones. Celebrate that you are doing it! Just knowing you need to start living healthier is a huge thing, as not many people are willing to admit to themselves that they need to lose some weight and eat healthier. Once you actually start doing it, that is even more amazing! You should be incredibly proud, and the continual encouragement will only help you achieve your goals much easier in the end.

If you do slip up and do something that goes against your diet and exercise plan, just look at it as a small loss and not a complete failure. By reminding ourselves that we just made a small mistake, we can find the courage to keep going. When we tell ourselves we failed and have to start over, it can be hard to get back on track. Accept that you are going to have small losses along the way and remember that you will have just as many small victories.

You Are Not Alone

Weight loss can be a lonely journey. It is up to us to get started, and we can only rely on ourselves to make sure that we follow through. It is likely that moments of loneliness are what led to our weight-loss struggles in the first place. Having to depend on just ourselves in this struggle can be what keeps us from achieving our goals. Sometimes, we are not strong enough to handle it all on our own, and that is okay. We need to remember that at first, we might need to ask for help. We shouldn't be expected to do it all by ourselves. When we become too dependent on ourselves for things that we can't always fix alone, there is a feeling of shame when we can't follow through.

When going through this journey, always remember that you are not alone. More than two in three adults are considered overweight. At this point, more people are struggling with their weight than those that are not. Even people that are not overweight still struggle with their perception of themselves as well as their overall body image. Don't be afraid to reach out and ask for help. Ask your parents for help in making sure they don't cook unhealthy meals or stock the fridge with junk food. Find a friend that also might be struggling with their weight and see if they want to start going on walks with you. The statistics prove that we are not in this alone, so there is no shame in reaching out for help.

One in thirteen adults have extreme obesity. When looking at weight-loss statistics like that, it is clear to see that you are certainly not alone in your weight-loss struggles. While these numbers might be concerning for our overall health and the way in which our society evaluates us, it can also be comforting to know that there are plenty people around us going through the same struggle. It is also a reminder that it is not our fault we got this way. We're certainly complicit in our own choices and can't blame the world for all of our health issues. It is a comforting reminder, however, to know that we're in a world set up for our weight issues. When a fast food meal is cheaper than a salad, we can't be so hard on ourselves when we do have moments of weakness.

Time Management

The most important part of a weight-loss journey is time management. This doesn't mean setting a quick goal and achieving it as fast as possible. It's all about using time properly and understanding how long it takes to actually do something. We set ridiculous goals for ourselves in the hopes that we'll achieve something great, but what ends up happening is, as the end-date approaches, we become overwhelmed and are set up for disappointment. We have to be realistic with our time goals and consider all factors when making different plans.

Practice Patience

Patience is hard to achieve. Anyone that wants to lose weight hopes that they can just jump on the scale after eating a salad and see the number drop by double digits. We have to accept before starting a weight-loss journey that this will never happen. We won't be able to just lose the weight overnight.

Sometimes, patience is hard to have when exercising. Many people find themselves getting bored on treadmills or other machines that require repetitive activity for minutes at a time. Use different exercise methods that you find fun or entertaining, such as a dance class or going on an interesting trail run. If the gym is your only option, use the boring moments on machines as a way to meditate. Clear your head, not thinking of how much weight you want to lose or what else you have to do to get there. Just practice counting or focusing on a quiet place you find peace in, such as a beach or a park. Visualize this in order to find a place of meditation. It'll take practice, but you'll soon find that you can zone out and work hard if you just focus.

There is No Rush

Weight loss takes time; we can't emphasize that enough. Some diets and exercises will help you lose weight quicker than others, but overall, you're going to have to put in a lot of time to lose weight. Remember not to feel too rushed throughout this journey. You have to be strict and consistent to actually see results, but there's no point in forcing yourself into ridiculous time constraints. If you cause yourself anxiety over certain dates, you might feel the need to stress-eat or go through dangerous dieting practices to get there.

Set Small Goals

Instead of looking at a wedding coming up in a couple of months as your goal for losing weight, instead, use that as a small milestone. Many of us get worried looking at the future, thinking of things coming up as the time limits for which we have to lose weight. Maybe it's March and you only have a couple months until swimsuit season. Instead of going on a diet to lose thirty pounds in three months, use the beginning of summer as a small milestone in your journey. Aim, instead, to be healthier and more confident by the time summer comes, rather than giving yourself a ridiculous goal that you don't even know if you can achieve.

Motivation-How to Make People Around You Help in Your Weight Loss Goals:

Let People Know About Your Goal

You should tell the people around you about your plan to lose weight. Most people will understand and adjust their behavior towards you. If they know that you want to lose weight, they are less likely to offer you foods you are avoiding and support you in your food choices. This will also help them understand why you have a different meal schedule.

Document and Track Your Progress

If you let the people around you see your progress, it will help them understand your point of view. Creating a blog or posting your personal weight loss victories on your social media accounts is a great way to motivate and keep you focused on your goals. Your friends that understand your goals will be supportive further boosting your motivation.

Hang Out with Supportive People

Surround yourself with people who share the same goals and concerns. You should find people who are also trying to lose weight. These are the types of people who congratulate you for your small victories and give you consoling words in the face of failure. They know how you feel because they are facing the same challenges. They will also be happy to have you around because your motivation also boosts theirs.

The following are tried and tested motivations to help keep you on the weight loss track.

Look for more than a single motivation

If there is one way to keep you motivated on your weight loss journey, it's to find more than just one single reason to stay motivated. Some of the motivations that you could use to make sure you stick to a healthy diet are:

Reaching Goal Weight

This all may seem kind of strict or a lot of information, but if you read it over and over again take the information in, it is actually simple. When you train your body to loosely follow these guidelines you can achieve weight loss. Every day is different and I am well aware that you cannot follow this regiment exactly and that is okay, but to have this guide to keep you grounded is helpful. You can master this concept and then adjust accordingly.

You will not eat much different when you reach your goal weight than when you eat while you are losing weight. What you are doing while you lose weight is simple not eating the junk that has put the weight on as well as you are nourishing your body with the proper foods so that it works efficiently.

Maintaining your own healthy weight means that you are watching what you eat and being conscious to eating good foods of the right portions so you feel good and look good.

Chapter 4: Gymnastics

How do smart women Exercise?

Some level of regular physical activity is a necessity for any successful weight loss program. Unfortunately, there is no way around it. You don't need to work out in a gym for two hours every day but you do need to have daily physical activity of at least 30-45 minutes. You simply cannot elevate your metabolism enough to lose weight without any exercise. There is no magic pill or potion that is going to make you achieve sustainable, healthy weight reduction without any exercise.

The healthiest time to exercise is two hours after a meal because your body has had time to digest your food and your blood can flow to your muscles instead of being diverted to your digestive tract to digest your food. The time that is most ideal for fat burning and quickly transforming your body is in the morning, before you have eaten any carbohydrates. This is because your body is coming out of a fasting state and it will have a lot of stored sugars for energy.

Your body will adapt if you engage in the same routine daily and lessen its beneficial effects. For instance, you can take a brisk walk, bicycle ride, use an elliptical machine, take a fitness class, do Pilates, yoga, or walk or run up and down an incline. The point is to try to vary your workout if possible, don't let your body adapt to the same daily regimen. Other great exercises are jumping rope, rowing, and circuit training in a gym.

Reasons Why You Should Exercise

- Dramatically increases your weight loss
- Build and tone muscle
- Increase your metabolic rate
- Increase your immune system's ability to combat disease
- Slow down aging and prevent osteoporosis
- Improve your mental outlook by looking and feeling better

How does yoga benefit women?

Practicing yoga can provide a woman with both expected and unexpected benefits in the mind, body and spirit. Yoga offers you joy, reflection, solace and acceptance of your body.

Yoga can help you to find balance, both physically and emotionally. It can help you to accept yourself, too. It aids in your physical balance, but also brings balance to your life, giving you a clearer perspective.

The postures of yoga are helpful in relieving stress and in losing weight more easily. Yoga allows you to connect with your inner self. You can work into a pose and be just yourself, listening to your breathing and appreciating what your body can do.

All Women Can Benefit from Yoga You can embrace yoga regardless of your age; it will support you wherever you are in life. Your yoga will evolve and become more complete as you age, becoming wiser and more intuitive.

With the pressures of daily life today, you will find support from other women who feel the same way as you about finding themselves and learning what is important to them.

Standing poses like the Tree Pose and Warrior Pose will help you find physical and emotional strength. The Camel Pose will help you in finding compassion and openness. The Corpse Pose and Child's Pose will give you a sense of being grounded in yourself.

PMS strains your body. You can use yoga poses to counteract those effects. Likewise, poses in yoga can help you deal with the changes in your body that come with menopause. Standing poses help to prevent bone loss and increase circulation during menopause.

Connecting to your Body Before yoga, you may never have connected with your body. This could be due to limited physical activity or a lack of self-acceptance. Yoga gives you a chance to use your body and mind, and opens up a new world for you, if you have not previously been accepting of yourself.

Yoga helps you to appreciate your own outer and inner beauty, allowing you to breathe, move and live. Yoga can assist you in appreciating the miracle of your body, where you can overcome negative habits and learn to love yourself.

Weight Loss Benefits of Yoga

There's a lot of work involved in losing weight. You have to pay close attention to your diet and all the things you eat and don't eat. You have to make sure you're getting enough exercise and burning more calories than you're eating. It can be all-consuming. Yoga can help you stay balanced and focused on the positive aspects of what you're doing, rather than the hard work and the deprivation. There are a number of ways that yoga can benefit your weight loss plans. Regular yoga practice treats your mind and your body. It burns calories and fat, gives your heart a cardio workout and brings an element of peace and mindfulness to your weight loss journey.

Body

Not a lot of people realize what a productive calorie burner yoga can be. It's not going to have you jumping and sweating like running, basketball or cross training. However, you do get a consistent calorie burn every time you dedicate 30 minutes or 60 minutes to yoga. Even a beginning yoga routine, with poses and positions found in Hatha yoga, allows you to burn around 300 calories in an hour. If you're going to pick up the pace a bit and do a more intense form of yoga such as Ashtanga or Vinyasa, you'll be able to burn even more. Movement of any kind provides the opportunity to burn calories.

The awareness of your body is another critical weight loss benefit when you're doing yoga. Each position and each pose requires you to focus on what your body is doing and how you are moving. You will be mindful of how the parts of your body work together and you'll be intimately in touch with each muscle and limb.

Flexibility is a huge benefit to doing yoga. All of the stretching you do will increase your balance and your ability to move. You'll notice your posture improves as well as the way you breathe and move. This might not seem like it would have an essential impact on losing weight, but it does. When you're able to move with more ease, your physical fitness level increases naturally. That keeps you moving and melting fat off your body. More flexibility means better fitness. You will notice that you look better in your clothes and you feel better when you are doing even simple things.

Mind

Yoga blends physical fitness with emotional and mental fitness. A large part of successful weight loss is positive thinking. When you incorporate a regular yoga practice into your weight loss strategy, you are training your mind to harness the power of intention and positivity. As you are stretching and holding poses, you can take the opportunity to visualize yourself as thinner, stronger and healthier. Existing in a state of expectation will help weight loss flow to you naturally. The mind is a powerful weapon in your weight loss battle and yoga will help you get in touch with that intention and put it to work for you.

Weight management is about managing stress as much as it's about cutting out the junk food and increasing the physical activity. When you get anxious or overwhelmed, your emotional imbalance can drive you towards bad habits. Yoga keeps you calm and trains you to lead yourself back to a state of peace when stress starts to invade your body and mind. That mindfulness will keep you balanced and positive.

Harnessing the Benefits

There are a number of practical ways to harness the weight loss benefits of yoga. When you're doing yoga, do it in a room without mirrors. A lot of yoga studios have mirrors, but try to avoid them. You want to remain positive and focused and if you're distracted by the sight of your thighs, you're disrupting your practice. Talk to yourself in positive terms. This will make you feel better about yourself and will also keep the entire weight loss process positive and not negative. Practice what's called "self-talk." As you're involved in yoga, talk to yourself with supportive words and motivational phrases. Be consistent with your yoga as well. Go to classes regularly or set aside a specific amount of time every day to focus on yoga.

Creating a better body does not have to be a struggle or a negative process. You can achieve dramatic weight loss results by making small buy meaningful changes to your life. One of those changes is yoga. In addition to eating well and exercising in a way that works for you, incorporate yoga and take advantage of the various physical and mental benefits that come with it. You'll continue losing weight and you'll also have a more positive, more mindful and more balanced outlook on your life and the body you're creating.

Select suitable sports to change your physique

I challenge you to change your perspective about exercise. For most people, saying the word "exercise" gives us the same queasy stomach feeling as "IRS, taxes, or lawyer." Instead of instantly imagining barbells, fitness clubs, and expensive personal trainers, consider another option. Consider being physically active, not necessarily exercising. When people decide they want to get healthier and lose some weight, they start by researching the newest and usually

50

expensive workout programs, local fitness facilities, and they also look online for expensive exercise equipment. Again, in order to make progress or show commitment most people feel like they need to lay some serious cash down to start the process. This is completely wrong. In fact, it is literally working against your success and results. I'm not saying personal trainers, gym memberships or buying workout programs and equipment won't help at all or can't be effective. What I'm saying is it is often unnecessary and expensive. After you've been active or working out for a month or two, you may feel ready to get more intense and focused on your activities or workouts. At that point, it makes complete sense to consider hiring someone to help or buying a program or product to move you forward with the habits you've already formed. My perspective is to start simple and low cost and only then should you proceed with getting more complicated and expensive. Find an activity such as a daily walk, bike ride or a light weight program you can do at home for free. Do this DAILY for a month or two to get your body used to the activity. This will help your endurance, flexibility, and strength while preventing injury. Also, the activity doesn't have to the same every day. Maybe one day you walk to the store and the next you ride your bike to a friend's house.

Stretching

Stretching is an awesome way to improve flexibility and prevent injury. There are a million different stretching programs available for free online. Also, yoga stretches and poses are very helpful to improve flexibility and reduce injury. Search for a PDF version of one designed by a medical clinic or physical therapy office, print it, and hang it up where you will be finishing your walk, light weight program or bike ride. Only stretch AFTER you are active. Never stretch much before being active. Muscles, tendons, ligaments and joints are not as flexible when they are cold.

Walking

By far the most effective habit for weight loss and to improve your overall health is to go for a daily walk.

The benefits are significant and if you start walking daily, you will experience a transformation in your health and quality of life. How can this be? It's because a brisk, daily walk gives you a good chunk of time to get away, relax, and enjoy some time to yourself. These days, having some time to yourself during the day is hard to find. Remember, the goal of any activity recommendations in this book is not to add yet another activity to your life but to get more value and benefit from the activities you already do.

Instead of committing to some expensive or complicated exercise regimen, just start going for a simple walk once a day. Take a family member or friend and go explore your neighborhood or community. Maybe make a habit that you can't have dinner or sit down to watch television or the computer until you've gone for your walk. Once you have done this for a month or so, this will become a habit and you'll look forward to it. At this point you will be able to decide what to do next. Do you go farther, faster, or maybe start lifting some weights? Do you decide to add some stairs or maybe riding a bike next time? It's really up to you but remember, you need to walk before you run!

Be sure to get your heart rate pumping a bit, maybe even a slight sweat and you'll know you are working hard enough. If you aren't able to talk while you are being active, then you are working too hard and need to dial it back a bit.

Our lifestyles have changed over time reducing the amount of activity we are getting both at work and at play. How many neighborhoods do you drive through in your town and see kids everywhere on their bikes and outside playing? It's very rare and ultimately the research reveals this is becoming a serious issue in our society as children are much less active and the rates of obesity and Type 2 diabetes in kids as young as ten years old are growing rapidly.

Running or Jogging

Before you start running, it is important that you make sure that running is the right option for you. There are certain factors that could put you at a higher risk for injury or other negative side effects: being over forty years of age, not accustomed to exercise, twenty pounds or more overweight, or a prior injury. If any of these factors apply, or if you have any concerns, consult your doctor before starting a running program.

Whether or not you consult with your doctor, you should still make sure to take it slowly when starting a running program. If you rush, you are likely to get discouraged, and possibly to injure yourself. Set a goal of being able to run continuously for thirty minutes – this will get you a great workout with a high level of calories burnt – but accept that it could take you quite a while to get there. Every person will go at his or her own pace. Set yourself reasonable goals; do not go too easy on yourself, but also do not expect too much.

In order to successfully implement running as part of your weight loss journey, you will need to schedule your workouts. Just like with taking the time to eat proper meals and snacks, if you do not take the time to get in a run then it is just not going to happen. You need to consciously commit the time to exercising. Put each workout into your calendar, or find some other way to make sure that you remember when you are supposed to go. And follow that schedule, regardless of the many excuses that you will likely be able to come up with as to why you should not, or do not, need to go running that day.

Try to start by running four minutes then walking for one minute; experiment to see what works for you. Gradually build up the time in which you can run continuously until you are able to run for the entire twenty minutes. Do not worry about how fast you are going; your speed will increase as you build up your stamina.

Pushups and Sit-ups

Start by doing a couple pushups and see you many you can do. Strive to do this several times daily and see how many you can do in a day! Try and do at least five of each exercise twice a day and soon it will be a habit which can make the difference in your upper body strength and core strength. If pushups are tough, start in a kneeling position instead of stretching out to balance on your toes, this is a bit easier and can help prevent injury as you are starting out. You can find some fun push-up and sit-up programs free online which can help you stay consistent. There is also at least one free app for your phone and tablet which will remind you and keep count of your pushups each day. Before long you'll be able to drop and give me twenty without even a sweat!

Treadmill and Riding Your Bike

Having a treadmill or stationary bike in your home is incredibly helpful for getting your daily activity completed. Based on that experience, you'll be able to decide how much you want to do the next day. The goal is to increase the time you are riding every week so you see progress. I recommend buying an inexpensive dry erase white board calendar and putting it up on the wall next to the treadmill or stationary bike. Write down either the time, distance or both of these each day and you'll see these numbers increase over time! It's very rewarding.

Weight lifting

Lifting weights is an incredible way to improve strength, flexibility, and endurance. Lifting weights can be completed with equipment at home or in the gym. Free weights or resistance bands seem to be the best and least expensive option. Using free weights and bands will also help build balance and coordination in your muscles to hold up a weight or perform reps correctly. Weight lifting machines can be used if you already have a gym membership however it's not necessary. There are tons of resources online to help you with starting a basic weight lifting program. Again, I recommend finding a cheap set of dumbbells, barbells, or resistance bands on Craigslist or some other local used site. Don't buy new unless you absolutely have to. Simply go online and you can find awesome sites with tons of helpful information. Stay away from any website which charges you a fee to use it or is trying to sell you something.

Swimming

Lap swimming, water aerobics and aqua classes are probably the easiest on your body of any exercises. That doesn't mean they're easy, it just means they aren't as tough on your body. Movement in water is easier on your joints and back than land-based exercise. Lap swimming is a great way to get aerobic exercise without the jarring effects of the ground. Even though it does require access to a swimming pool, it doesn't require much else besides a swimsuit, goggles and a swim cap. Most fitness facilities with pools generally provide relatively inexpensive swim lessons and classes on how to swim if you need to learn or hone your skills. Water-based aerobics classes aren't just for grandmas anymore. Many wellness centers even offer sessions where yoga is performed on paddle boards. Don't rush out and pay for an expensive gym membership just to use the pool. If you already have a membership, that's great. But if not, keep your cash and just start with the other forms of activity for now.

Simple Sleep Truth

Sleep, Sleep, Sleep there is nothing that will help you weight loss more than the right amount of sleep and rest. You cannot make any excuse for this. Some people get by on little sleep when they are younger and stay thin, if this is not you then you have a different type of body. You have to rearrange everything you do in order to sleep on a schedule and have a rhythm that your body can count on.

You can step outside the schedule once a week, but otherwise your body looks for repetition to make it feel safe and rested. Everything you think you do when you do not get enough sleep can be done with enough sleep. It just becomes a matter of rearranging your schedule to fit everything in.

A great sleep pattern is to go to bed around 9 or 10 and get up at about 5 or 6 am. At first you might be a little resistant if you have not usually been sleeping on this schedule.

A really bad thing is to sleep strange times and different amounts on a regular basis.

The right amount of sleep helps you have the proper emotional state of mind. Sleep is when the body repairs itself. Sleep keeps your natural system working the way it is supposed to for proper immune system function.

Mixing Weight Loss and Socializing

Deciding to eat healthier and watching your caloric intake does not mean that you need to give up socializing and eating out. At first, it may be easier to stick with your amended diet if you are avoiding negative influences and the temptation of high-calorie restaurant meals, but you do not need to avoid it forever.

The first thing that you need to accept is that you will be faced with temptation, and you will need to overcome it. Restaurants are in the business of offering delicious food and accompanying drinks, and for the most part, those menu items are not going to fit into your reduced calorie diet. Knowing your options will help you to resist temptation and ensure that your meal stays in line with your caloric limits, while still tasting great.

If possible, check out the restaurant online and see if they have an online menu. If you have an idea ahead of time of some of the more nutritious, low-calorie meal options, it will be easier to order that meal when the time comes rather than making the decision while your friends are all ordering the less-healthy meals.

One area where the calories add up faster than you would believe is drinks, especially when it comes to alcohol. In addition to being high in calories, most drinks are empty calories only: lots of calories with little to no nutritional value. Order water whenever possible – yes, it may be less fun and less tasty, but you can spend your calories elsewhere and still get some nutrition out of it, which is just not going to happen with drinks.

When selecting the entrée that you are going to order, choose options that include the words grilled, boiled, or roasted. Entrées prepared in this way tend to be lower in calories and fat. Try to avoid fried foods completely – you would be amazed at how quickly the calories add up when you are eating fried foods! If you are ordering a pasta dish, select a tomato-based sauce rather than a cream-based one, as that will be much lower in calories. For side dishes, choose steamed vegetables (without butter), a baked potato (hold the butter and sour cream), or plain rice.

When it comes to dessert, avoiding it is, of course, the best option. If you do decide that you need to have something, try a fruit cup or sorbet if it is available. If you go with something heavier, see if someone else at your table will split it with you – that will let you have a taste of the dessert without eating all of the calories.

The most important thing to remember when you are eating out with your friends or family is that if you eat in moderation, you will be able to stick to your diet and still enjoy your socializing. You do not need to deny yourself everything, and you should not do so because you will be less likely to stick to the diet if you constantly feel that you deny yourself. But you also should not go all-out and order whatever you want, because, in addition to that meaning that you will go over your caloric allowance, it could also have the impact of making you feel like you have failed, which could increase the likelihood of you giving up. Moderation is key.

All of this will help you when it comes to picking which foods to order when you are out eating with your friends or family, but what do you do when your eating partners encourage you to give in to temptation?

You need to make it clear to them ahead of time that you will be working to stick within your caloric allowance, and that you need them to support you in making this decision and resisting temptation. If the people with whom you intend to socialize indicate that they will not be supporting you, or do not take your request seriously, then you should think twice before you go out with them. It is a lot easier to resist temptation when the people around you are encouraging and supporting you.

How to set up your smart exercise schedule

Dieting helps set the pace for weight loss while exercising keeps up the momentum. There is no smooth weight loss without adding at least 30 minutes of exercising. It is quite easy to ignore working out and concentrate on dieting because you feel that there is no time or even energy to get on the treadmill or go to the gym.

It may be difficult and daunting to engage in working out while cutting calories, but if you focus on the goal which is losing weight, you will scale through it. Moreover, you only need 30 minutes aerobic or resistant exercise to get the fats burning.

One importance of exercise while shedding fat is that it increases your metabolism making it easier to lose weight. When dieting, there is a stage you will get to, called a plateau. It's when your body begins to adapt to the new style of eating and exercise, make losing weight difficult. This can be corrected through exercise and different levels of resistance training which will help in increasing your metabolism and get you out of that plateau.

Before engaging in any exercise, it is safer to check with your doctor if you have any health risk like high blood pressure or high blood sugar so that you do not have complications. There are different exercises you can engage in, all you need to do is have your exercise routine and stick to it. You can start by walking if it's your first time exercising or you've not done so in a while.

Walking helps you to burn fat over time, especially belly fat. It also helps in preserving lean muscles mass and helps in stress management, one of the causes of weight gain.

You can include walking into your exercise routine by walking to work if your office or business place is close to home. If not, you can use the public transport, stop a bus stop away and walk to wherever you are going. Also, use the stairs rather than the elevator and use your legs rather than your car or public transports when running errands close to you. And while walking, ensure that you engage your arms and walk briskly.

From walking, you can progress to jogging, swimming, running, and then resistant training. Resistance training will help improve metabolism, increase your lean muscle mass which helps lower your fat mass. You can increase your level of resistance every month to keep up your metabolism rate. Examples of resistance training are pushups, mountain climbing, planking, weight lifting, *etc.*

If you notice it's difficult to get motivation to exercise each day, you can get a gym membership or an exercise buddy. Get new gym kits to make your subconscious mind feel your eagerness to change the course of your life.

How to Keep It Going

Losing weight is not the easiest thing to do, and I know that it can be a challenge. The key to any successful weight loss program is to keep a positive mental attitude and know beyond a shadow of a doubt that YOU CAN DO IT! Take a second to really think about this new path that you are on and congratulate yourself. Be happy. I have given you the keys to succeed but it is your turn to take the knowledge you have just obtained and put it into use!

But before I go, let me leave you with one last tip.

There are the two main factors that are essential in achieving anything in life. Your surroundings and mindset. If you surround yourself with positive, goal-oriented, passionately healthy people, you will become a positive, passionately fit and healthy person. Who you surround yourself with is who you will become. In order to succeed in any long term fat loss program, you are going to have to make serious changes and really think about the circles that you keep. If your friends and family eat poorly, you need to let them know that having those foods around hurts your chance at success. You have to KNOW that you are a healthy individual with not only the ability to lose more weight, but the ability to keep it off and live a healthy lifestyle. You have to know that this is not only a possibility, but an actuality.

Keeping the Weight Off

The part where many people really fall through with their goals is after they actually achieve them! Many people get to their desired weight, see that number, and think they no longer have to keep up with their diet plan. Then, the weight comes back, and the cycle of disappointment has to be lived all over again. Remember that once you reach your first goal, you should set another one. The second might not be as extreme. For example, maybe your first goal is to get down to 180 pounds. Once you do that, you have to come up with something new. That might be getting down to 170 pounds, or it could be something different, such as improving the muscle mass in a certain part of your body. Never stop setting goals. The level of difficulty can fluctuate. But to stay on track and keep the weight off, you have to continually encourage yourself to do better.

Change Things Up

Some people might find that after a year or two of dieting and exercising, they stop losing weight. This can be because their bodies are now used to the healthy behavior. You probably won't ever lose as much weight in a diet as you do at the beginning. Those transformations can be invigorating, but remember that as you continue, it will become a little less drastic.

If you feel you've plateaued in your diet, you should consider changing things up. This might involve trying an entirely new diet, or it could be working out in a different way. Incorporating variety helps to ensure that you'll stick to your goals while also having fun!

Take it Slowly

You will need to learn how to prepare food in a different way, how to eat more vegetables and fruits, maybe even how to shop properly and your body is going to react hard to a sudden change. It needs to learn how to digest these new foods and how to stop craving addictive foods for a start. The harder your body reacts, the more likely you are to give it all up so the best thing to do is ease yourself in. Give your mind and your body a chance to adjust to your new way of life and you will be more likely to hang on to the motivation to succeed. Keep this in mind – it doesn't matter how fast you make changes, what matters is that you do and you stick with them for the long term.

Find treats and comfort foods that are healthy

When you first make the change to a healthy diet, you might feel a little lost. The simple reason for that is that you are used to eating your favorite treats and those comfort foods you turned for in times of need and you are feeling a bit empty and as if there's a big void that needs to be filled. There are plenty of healthy treats and comfort foods that can fill that void. If you have a sweet tooth and tend to turn to chocolate, simply puree up a banana and some cocoa powder with some ground flax to make a healthy chocolate pudding.

Keep things simple

You don't need to prepare complicated gourmet meals every day. Yes, it is nice to take time over preparing a meal and making it look good but for most meals you can stick to basic foods, like steamed vegetables and rice, a baked sweet potato or a soup. Just use those herbs, spices and vinaigrettes I talked about earlier to spice things up in simple ways. Find meals that you really enjoy and just make a few simple changes to keep them interesting.

64

Never feel guilty

It takes time to make the transmission from an unhealthy diet to a healthy one and it is important that you do not get obsessive over what you are doing. Stress causes an awful lot of problems health-wise and it is important that you do not stress yourself out over what you eat. Nobody can stick to a healthy diet every single day; we all have days where we give in to temptation. Guilt is a negative emotion and they simply make you eat more to feel better about yourself. Don't punish yourself by eating less or exercising harder and longer because that won't work either. Simply take each day as it comes and move on. If you slip up, simply pick yourself back up and carry on with your new healthy diet.

Stay positive

Positive energy is the key to realizing your goals. Unfortunately, most people tend to focus so much energy on avoiding the bad stuff that they miss out on the fun of trying new foods and the effects that a good nourishing diet has on your body. Find healthy foods that you love to eat, like fruits, some nuts, or a special healthy dinner. Eat them as often as you can so that maintain a positive attitude and keep that positive energy flowing through you.

Knowing this will be the biggest factor in your success. You have to know that you are choosing the right items to put in your body and that you are moving and exercising enough to burn calories.

This is who you are and this is what you do. You are healthy and you are fit and you are happy! Losing weight is equally mental as it is physical, but I know you can do it. You can go out into the world as a fresh new person, and a newer, healthier, fitter you!

How Being Overweight Affects Your Mind?

Anyone can have a fit body, but that doesn't always mean they have a healthy mind. Mental illness like bipolar disorder, depression, and anxiety have the ability to affect many different people, no matter their size. With that in mind, it is also important to know that being overweight can have some seriously negative effects on your brain. Someone that struggles with mental illness and who is overweight might find that shedding some pounds actually improves their overall mental health as well.

Those who are overweight have issues with depression and anxiety more often than physically fit individuals. Part of this is because of the way society treats overweight individuals. When thin models are plastered all over billboards and other advertisements, it can be hard to not have a warped perception of bodies that don't look the same as those airbrushed beauties. However, more so than just the way our society affects body image, there are physical effects being overweight has on the brain.

Being overweight might lead to a higher risk of getting Alzheimer's or dementia. This is partially because excess weight affects the hippocampus, which we'll discuss in the next section. The foods that we eat, and how much oxygen we're giving our body, increase and decrease certain chemical levels in our brain which, in turn, may cause mental illnesses and disorders. These can end up leading to more weight loss on top of that as well.

There is a "dulling" effect on those who are overweight which leads to less enjoyment and pleasure from eating certain foods. When we drink sugary drinks all day, we become used to that constant sugar intake. This ends up warping our perception on sugary sweets, which means we get used to them and end up wanting more. In order to understand how this dulling effect works, start by giving up just one food you eat all the time. Before you start with a full-on diet, just give up something "bad for you" that you eat a few times a week, such as a sugary Starbucks drink, a nightly candy bar, a morning donut, or anything else that you consistently eat that is sweet. After just a week free of your item of choice, go ahead and indulge. You will be shocked at how sweet it might taste. This is because you have reduced your tolerance. You might find that the pleasure from just that one drink is so much greater than the consistent level of gratification you get from giving into your frequent indulgence.

The striatum is a part of our brain that is responsible for pleasure regulation. In overweight individuals, especially women, the striatum becomes weakened, giving us less pleasurable responses. This means that in terms of more than just food, we'll receive less pleasure from things that normally would bring us great joy. By eating healthier and exercising regularly, we're also taking care of our striatum which means our pleasure levels will rise back to where they should be. This is pleasure in all forms, whether it is from food, family, friends, music, sex, or anything else that brings us joy and happiness. The healthier our striatum, the more pleasure we'll feel.

Chapter 5: Ketogenic Diet and Weight Loss for Women

Ketogenic diet is a diet that places and trains your body to be in a state wherein it primarily uses fat for energy. It achieves this through a natural metabolic process of your body called Ketosis that uses fat to create fuel for your body. A ketogenic diet has many similarities to the Atkins diet and many other low-carb diets. It has been known by several different names like low carb high fat, low carb diet and of course, the ketogenic diet.

The ketogenic diet can be implemented by discarding most of the sugars and starches in your diet and by eating healthy fats, moderate amounts of protein and very low carbs. With little carbohydrates in your diet, your body does not receive enough glucose to keep up with your body's caloric requirements. This eventually results in decreasing blood sugar levels in your body as it uses up glucose for its functions. When you eat foods that are high in carbs, your body automatically produces insulin and glucose. Insulin is made to process the glucose that is in your bloodstream by moving it around the body. Glucose is easy for your body to convert and be used for energy. Therefore, it gets chosen over all other energy sources.

As blood sugar level decreases, it looks for the stored glycogen present in your body and breaks it down to glucose and dissolves it in your blood to be distributed throughout your body. However, glycogen stores would also eventually run out. And when it does, your body would start to use fats as a source of energy for functions in its different parts and produce ketones when the liver processes it. Since glucose is used as the primary energy source, the fat in your body isn't needed and gets stored. With a normal, high carb diet, your body uses glucose as its main form of energy. By lowering the carb intake, the body is put into ketosis. These fats could come from the food that you eat, from your meals or from the fat that your body stores. This is what is called ketosis.

When you hit ketosis, your body starts being very efficient at burning fat to create energy. It turns fat in the liver into ketones that supply energy to the brain. Many studies have shown that a keto diet can help you to improve your health and lose some weight. It can also help with Alzheimer's disease, epilepsy, cancer and diabetes.

The primary advantage of following a ketogenic diet is that it restores the capability of your body to use both fat and glucose as fuel to meet its energy or caloric needs. Your body is designed to use both glucose and fat as fuel. However, due to eating a high carbohydrate diet for most of their lives, many people lack the ability to use fat for the body's energy needs. This results in bodies that have a hard time maintaining a healthy weight and a healthy body fat percentage, both of which contribute to poor health. In fact, even if you are not overweight or obese, you may still have excess visceral fat, which is wrapped around your organs like your liver, pancreas and kidneys.

With a ketogenic diet, your body restores its flexibility to use both glucose and fat as fuel for its energy needs. This flexibility keeps your fat cells, both visceral and subcutaneous (the fat located under your skin and on top of your muscles), in check by using the stored energy found in those fat cells. This would, in turn, reduce the risks of having diseases involved with having high-fat stores, specifically visceral fat:

- Type 2 Diabetes
- Coronary Artery/ Heart Disease
- Colorectal Cancer
- Breast Cancer
- High Cholesterol
- High Blood Pressure
- Metabolic Syndrome
- Alzheimer's Disease
- Stroke
- Dementia

Other than decreasing risks of said diseases, this flexibility contributes to losing excess fat and weight in a manageable manner. Normally, while and after losing some weight, your body would feel less sated after eating the same meal you ate before the weight loss process started.

And in addition to this, you might feel an increase in appetite to compensate especially if you've been depriving yourself. However, when your body is in a state of ketosis, ketones help your body manage the hormones that decrease your satiety after meals and increase your appetite and hunger. With this, you lose weight without fighting your body to gain it back through its natural responses as to what it believes to be starvation.

Moreover, being able to utilize glucose and fat for energy prevents you from experiencing the big swings that affect your mental focus, making you hungry and irritable. When glucose runs out, ketones are readily available to fuel your brain. Even better, ketones give your brain a boost, enabling you to have better focus and concentration.

Your body undergoes some changes or adjustments when you start the keto diet. You may feel dizzy, a bit irritable, feel fatigued, or have a headache, but do not fret for these are just normal symptoms saying your body is adjusting. Stick with the diet, and you will be alright since your body is just undergoing withdrawal from carbohydrates and sugar. However, it is always vital to visit your doctor and undergo consultation before going into these kinds of diets.

As your body undergoes such adjustments, it is imperative that you drink lots of water. Water helps in relieving all those symptoms you are feeling. The objective of the keto diet is not to starve you, but in lowering down the intake of carbohydrates in your body, you allow your body to adapt to whatever you put into it. So, if you put in more fats over carbs, it will burn ketones, or those fats, making them your body's source of energy....and you will be fine!

Your body may be adjusting to this type of diet, but you will be surprised how energized you will get. Thus, this provides you with a clearer state of mind, enabling you to think clearer. Your sleeping patterns will improve as well as decrease your joint pains and illness of your muscles.

Ketogenic diet provides great improvements in the lives of those patients with medical conditions stated above. Overall, the keto diet is very beneficial to all by helping individuals achieve healthier lives. On the other hand, it is important also to note that if you have Type1 diabetes, this type of diet is not advisable for your condition. You must first ensure that your blood sugar is stable or in a normal state. Please be guided and still follow the recommendations of your physician.

A list of foods allowed on the ketogenic diet.

- Fish, except for farmed fish, or fish certified with the Marine Stewardship Council. The safest species: salmon, red salmon, anchovy, herring, sardines. Try to avoid fish fried with olive oil (oil for packing of fish is not for human consumption).

- Meat: lamb, pork, poultry meat (free-range chicken), game, meat preparations, beef (pasture-fed cow). Moderate consumption of bacon and sausages is also allowed.

- Vegetables: asparagus, avocado, broccoli, brussels sprout, white cabbage, cauliflower, celery, cucumbers, kale cabbage, mushrooms, green salad, greens sauté, spinach, zucchini.

- After your body is readjusted for fat burning, you can return a restricted amount of vegetables to your diet, such as eggplant, garlic, onion, parsnip, pepper, turnip, tomatoes, pumpkin (small amount).

- Fruit and berries: a little handful of any berries to substitute vegetables, some grapefruit wedges to substitute vegetables.

By following the above-suggested list, you will be able to devise an individual meal plan. In addition, it is important to count calories and not to exceed the permissible norm. Observing simple rules will contribute to having a beautiful body and a feeling of well-being.

Foods to avoid on the ketogenic diet.

- Factory-processed fats – vegetable oils (sunflower oil, rape oil, peanut oil, cottonseed oil, corn oil, soy oil);
- Trans fats – salad dressings from food stores, mayonnaise, peanut oil and other products containing hydrogenated fats;
- Milk and cottage cheese, kefir, yoghurt, ricotta (high-protein products);
- Sugar;
- Ketchup, salsa, BBQ sauce, soy and tomato sauce;
- Juice, smoothie from food stores;
- Sweet white and sparkling wine;
- Any cereals;
- Bananas, apples and other restricted fruit;
- Grapes;
- Bread;
- Cakes;
- Potato;
- Pastry.

Any high-carbohydrate products are to be avoided. When consumed, they cause the liver to produce glycogen that does not produce ketone bodies. Even a little excess of carbohydrates can reduce all efforts to zero and fill the body with more fat cells. It is important to read the contents of all purchased products carefully: even common seasoning may contain unfavorable starch or sugar.

Hazards of the Ketogenic diet and Contraindications.

As with any diet, a keto meal plan alters the body. Everyone is individual and reacts to new nutritional habits in a specific way. Not giving up is important, as the first tangible results will not come immediately.

Major side effects may include the following:

- Dehydration — a simple way out is to drink more water. Sipping slightly salted chicken, fish or beef broth is also allowed.

- Nausea – start taking digestive supplements such as pancreatine to aid digestion.

- Confused mental state – it is caused by lack of glucose in the first days on the diet, which is only temporary.

- Gastrointestinal tract abnormalities - consume more dietary fiber (nuts, flax seeds) and water to avoid troublesome pain from constipation.

75

- Fatigue and general discomfort - reduced amounts of glucose in your blood may cause you to become tired easily. Check your carnitine levels and replete it if necessary.

- Muscle cramps – try taking salt baths and vitamin K2 to increase your electrolyte levels.

In the early stages of the diet, the absence of glucose causes drowsiness, irritation, reduced mental alertness and activity. Each of these unpleasant feelings is gone within a week after starting the diet. This is the time for your body to get used to and adapt to the new conditions. Not giving up and ensuring you only consume allowed foods is essential.

Consult your doctor before starting the ketogenic diet.

Basics of Planning Meals

To know what you have to eat on a ketogenic diet, you will have to understand caloric requirements and content and fats, protein and carbohydrates. You have to understand their different kinds and the different roles they perform for your body. Furthermore, you need to know what macronutrients are good and harmful for your health so that you can build a diet that is both ketogenic and healthy.

In addition, for the ketogenic diet to work, you need to remove all packaged and processed foods from your diet. It should consist of high-quality, healthy fats, fiber-rich carbohydrates with the least net carbohydrates (total carbohydrates minus fiber) as possible.

Important: Before you create a plan for your ketogenic diet, you need to consult first a nutritionist or a medical professional to determine the number of daily calories you require based on your age, height, weight, gender and age as well as body fat percentage. This would make sure that you are not merely guessing in setting the calories you need for your body.

Fats

Fats in your diet contain mixtures of fatty acids. These nutrients contain a mixture of saturated and unsaturated fats. Saturated fats are most abundant in animal-derived fats while unsaturated fats are most abundant in plant-derived ones. Other than the dense caloric property fats, it provides fatty acids that regulate inflammation in the body. It carries fat-soluble vitamins. Lastly, it provides texture and flavor to your meal, making it more satisfying to your appetite.

Proteins to eat

Moderate consumption of high-quality protein is the key. Protein for a ketogenic diet should come from a variety of plant and animal sources. Meat products should be lean to avoid adding fats that are mostly saturated. The suggested protein for a ketogenic diet varies from person to person. Generally, the recommended daily protein of 0.8g per pound of lean body mass for a sedentary lifestyle, 0.8 to 1g per pound of body mass for a lightly active lifestyle and 1.0 − 1.2g for a highly active lifestyle.

Carbohydrates

Carbohydrates are the starches, sugars and fibers found in the food that we eat. The sugars and starches we eat are broken down into its simplest chemical forms while, as it is indigestible, fibers just pass through the digestive system.

Sugars, also known as simple carbohydrates, are found in fruit and vegetables that can be broken down to sucrose and/ or fructose. Starches, also known as complex carbohydrates, are found in grains that can be broken down into glucose (also known as blood sugar).

Of all these carbohydrates, glucose is the most preferred as it can be readily circulated from the digestive process into various parts of the body. Meanwhile, fructose can only be used for energy by the liver and sucrose is further broken down into glucose and fructose.

The role of fiber: The most common question with low carb dieters is: Do I need to include fiber when counting my carbs?

Let's see: Some soluble gets absorbed, but humans, in general, don't possess all the needed enzymes to digest fibers and then be able to get calories out of it. Because of this, fiber doesn't affect blood sugar or ketosis. You can try to get between 20 and 25 grams of net carbs or less than 50 grams of total carbs.

If the fiber isn't counted, the carbs are referred to as net carbs. Calculating net carbs can reduce how high fiber foods are impacted and allow you to eat them. This is a common argument for those who criticize the low carb diet because it lacks fiber. An important note is that fiber does not negate carbs. They are just not counted. You can't just mix some flax meal into pasta.

Fibers also contain phytochemicals like lycopene, lutein and indole-3-carbinol. These stimulate the immune system, fight free radicals and protect and repair the DNA.

Why the Ketogenic Diet Is Effective for Weight Loss

The body's chemistry, not the arithmetic of calories in versus calories out, is what determines whether people gain weight or lose weight. Consuming carbs leads to the production of insulin, which turns on the body's fat-producing hormones. Research is increasingly finding that insulin is directly related to weight gain. Unless you immediately burn off the sugars that you consume, they will be stored as fat. This occurs regardless of whether you are eating "diet" foods or not. The key to losing weight is not in restricting calories but in lowering your insulin levels.

People on the ketogenic diet often find that they lose weight without having to restrict calories. They feel less hungry, have a much more stable appetite and feel more satisfied after eating. Without sugar being used as the body's primary fuel source, they immediately begin to burn through fat.

The ketogenic slim down additionally works since it is satisfying. As prior said, a ketogenic count calorie is high in fat, adequate protein and low in carb. Fats are satisfying as are proteins. In this way, you will feel full for more and have no compelling reason to indulge.

The ketogenic consume fewer calories additionally works since it enacts fat digestion on account of the decreased level of insulin in the body. Given that you decline your admission of carbs, your blood has less of glucose, which implies that there won't be a requirement for the discharge of high measures of insulin. Remember that other than encouraging the cells to ingest glucose, insulin has the impact of repressing fat digestion (lipolysis). Preferably, it advances fat stockpiling and glycogen collection (glycolysis). With decreased insulin levels, your body can adequately begin utilizing fats since there is no hindrance. You can read more here and here.

With that comprehension of the ketogenic count calories, let us now look top to bottom at what precisely happens to your body when on a ketogenic consume fewer calories.

Ketogenic Diet Plan

Let set a 7-day Ketogenic diet plan for starting your journey. You can take it as the first test and know what kind of Ketogenic diet plan suits you the most. It is useless if you do not know your own body and understand what is Ketogenic diet in reality.

For more Ketogenic diet recipes – highly recommend you read my book "7-day Keto diet meal – fresh and healthy keto instant pot recipes cookbook" in my page at Amazon to find your Keto recipes – it is easy to follow and help you lead a healthy lifestyle.

Diet Challenges That Make Women Hate Losing Weight

Fear

One of the biggest challenges is fear. You can avoid fears strengthening yourself, identifying and facing them. Most types of modern fears are all in the mind and only succeed in making us avoid new experiences. This is the nature of modern types of fear.

Not all fears are bad however. Some of them are rational and warn us that our life may be in danger if we carry on with what we are doing and others that have nothing to do with survival at all.

Identify your fears, and separate the ones that are rational from the ones that are unnecessarily paralyzing us.

Put yourself in experiences where you can face them. These experiences will desensitize you from the factors that you fear. As your mind becomes accustomed to working with these factors, it will no longer generate the sensation of fear every time you are about to face the same experience.

Paralyzing Self-Perception

Sometimes fear lead to a distorted way of seeing ourselves. If you think that you are incapable of reaching fitness goals then you have sabotaged yourself from reaching success. You have surrendered even before starting the battle.

First accept it. The usual reaction when someone points this out to them is denial. You tend to deny that your self-perception is the main factor that prevents you from even signing up to the gym or creating a diet plan.

Second, build your self-esteem by winning personal victories. Personal victories are the foundations of a healthy self esteem. You could start by taking on small weight loss related tasks and if achieve success with these tasks, write them down in a list. As the list of your personal victories become longer, you will become more confident to take on more difficult tasks.

How Others Look at You

Some people fear of being judged by others affects their actions too much. They don't follow the plan in times when their mind becomes occupied by how other people think of them. They are prone to over eating when they are together with a group who makes fun of their attempt to lose weight.

People around YOU can be mean. They ridicule YOU for trying to lose weight because of your own failure to do so. They make you feel horrible because deep inside that's how they feel with their own weight and health problems. Most fit people like to talk about how they remain fit because they are self-centered but also because many of them like to motivate others to do the same. A fit person feels bad every time they see someone they love suffering from weight issues.

Extreme Stress

If your mind is pre-occupied with important thoughts they cause you to become stressed out, you may not have the focus to continue on your workout and diet plan.

You could deal with the cause of your stress first before continuing to work out. Or you could try to stick to your plan even in the face of great mental stress.

How to Boost Your Motivation to Maintain Your Diet Plan?

People usually eat more than their fair share when they haven't planned their food source for the day. Office workers are prone to this problem. They are usually absorbed in their jobs and they don't give a lot of thought on the sources of their foods. This makes them reliant on unhealthy food sources like preserved food products or fast food.

You can avoid these sources of foods by planning out your meals throughout the day. You will have a stronger chance of resisting temptations of food if you are not hungry most of the time. To do this, you should evenly space your meal throughout the day.

The ideal meal plan is to eat 6 small meals in your waking hours. Most adults eat 3 big meals and countless snacks in between. After eating one of their big meals, they will probably feel hungry again after 2 hours. Because it is not yet time for another big meal, they snack on the available food sources around them. For most people, the basis for their food choices is the taste. Tasty foods are usually high in fats and calories. You can avoid choosing these by creating a weekly meal plan.

Keep in mind that we are trying to avoid those instances where you need to rely on preserved and fast foods in your meals and snacks. To do this, you will need to prepare your own food each day. It is highly suggested to prepare your food for the whole day every morning. You should follow the daily prescribed amount of calories when preparing your meals. The next step is to divide the food that you prepare into six and place them into vacuum sealed containers to preserve their freshness.

The average person is awake for 16 hours a day. That means that you should eat your meals every 2 and a half to 3 hours. If you want to avoid eating before you sleep, you could modify the process by eating only five times a day. You will eat slightly bigger meals but the amount of calories that you take in will still be the same.

By following this plan, you will reduce the amount of calories that you take in at one time. Your body will have more time to digest the foods that you take in and by the time you eat your next meal, your body will have already digested the majority of the previous meal.

Because your meals are evenly spaced, you will not become hungry in between meals. This will lessen your unhealthy snacking and prevent you from relying on fast foods and high-calorie packaged foods. You will be satisfied most the time, which means that you will have stronger will power to resist offers of food.

How intelligent women lose weight in a short Time-Mindfulness Training Helps

When a person is conscious of their surroundings and what their eating habits might be, they are more aware of the factors that make up for the fundamentals of why they are eating. Mindfulness is an attempt at a person putting emphasis on their surroundings and what's physically happening at any given time. Mindfulness is all about not thinking of the future or ruminating about the past. Reminiscing and planning are not harmful, but doing too much of either thing can certainly be.

Maintaining a diet can be the biggest problem for those who embark on a weight-loss journey. When a person is mindful, they will better be able to control their current situation instead of worrying so much about the past or future. When a person is mindful, they can better control their own thoughts and emotions rather than feeling overwhelmed by all their thoughts. If someone is always anxious about the future, they are going to be very worried about keeping up with their diet. They are taking on feelings of future failure instead of focusing on how to actually prevent that failure in the present moment. When we're not mindful, it can lead to moments of stress and anxiety that will lead to overeating or punishment purging.

The biggest way to be mindful about eating is to not do it while you are doing something else. Instead of sitting down in front of the TV, try to eat at a table where you can talk to someone else. If you focus on the show rather than how much you are eating, you are likely to continually stuff yourself until you are in pain rather than carefully tracking how much you are eating. You might grab a bag of chips when a movie starts, and before you know it, you are only halfway through the movie but all the way through the bag. The best way to be mindful when you eat is to just focus on only eating. This can be more enjoyable when meals are shared as well.

Appreciate the food that you are eating. In order to practice mindful eating, take in every bite slowly and focus on how it makes you feel overall rather than on what you might be doing later. Taste the food and savor each bite. Think of the work that went into creating that meal and the positive effects the food is going to have on your body. When we put an emphasis on this rather than on other things, we eat much slower which means we end up digesting better.

Sometimes, we eat so fast that we still feel hungry, so we end up going back for more. Instead, eat slowly so that you can feel yourself getting full rather than just trying to eat as much as possible. Take a break in between portions in order to ensure you are not just eating because you can. If you eat a lot of food in a quick amount of time, you are just setting yourself up for a night of misery.

Not only does this help someone in their weight-loss journey, but it can have very positive effects on other areas of one's life as well. Being mindful is not important just to shed pounds. It is also crucial to making sure you are actually living in the moment and enjoying your surroundings. Sometimes, eating might be a way to distract ourselves from different forms of pain. If we're mindful of that pain and how to overcome it, we're not only better off in our life in general, but we also eliminate the urge to eat when we aren't hungry.

Long-Term Tips

No matter how much you love the ketogenic diet, there are family reunions, parties and other events that can easily derail your best-laid plans. Holidays and birthdays can be particularly difficult, as you are surrounded by sweet and savory dishes that bring back fond memories. Being surrounded by relatives and friends who lovingly prepared all of the food can make resisting even more difficult. Having to prepare food separately from what you feed your family can be difficult. Additionally, you are probably finding that the ketogenic diet takes a lot of commitment. Food preparation, storage and grocery shopping can take vastly larger amounts of time than before. Plus, it costs more than eating a high-carb diet. Here are some tips to help you stay on the ketogenic diet long-term.

Plan ahead

Planning your meals in advance is a strategic way to manage a busy schedule while sticking to a healthy eating plan. Prepare your grocery list before you go to the store so that you don't forget anything that you need. Having to make an extra grocery trip during the week can easily cost you an hour or two.

Make sure that you always have keto-friendly foods on you. Invest in some food containers that you can easily put in your bag and take with you places. Keep them filled with things like nuts, vegetable sticks, yogurt dip and sliced avocados. At a sports game, in a meeting, out on a long shopping excursion, or anytime that you have to be away from home for more than a few hours, you can pop the containers out and recharge on ketogenic foods.

One challenge of the ketogenic diet is that many foods have to be eaten immediately after being prepared. The thought of eating scrambled eggs that have been in the refrigerator for a couple of days is less than appetizing. Look for recipes that can be prepared in advance and eaten throughout the week. Examples include curries, soups and casseroles. Take one day each week to prepare some dishes that can be refrigerated and eaten throughout the week. This will save you a lot of time and enable you to stay on track, even on your busiest days.

Know what local restaurants have keto-friendly options on their menus so that when you do go out to eat, you already know what you can order without derailing your diet. Just because something isn't labeled keto-friendly doesn't mean that it isn't. An omelet with cheese is probably fine, as long as you don't add hash browns or anything else on the side. If you are at a restaurant that doesn't have anything that appears to be keto-friendly, ask for something to be specially prepared, based on the ingredients that appear in the other foods on the menu. For example, if there are choices that contain avocados, cucumbers and oil and vinegar dressing, you can request that those ingredients be made into a salad.

Take advantage of grocery delivery

Grocery shopping can be a time-consuming hassle, but nowadays, many stores offer grocery delivery. You select online what you want and when you want it to be delivered, then pay online via credit or debit card. This can shave hours every week off of the time you spend on maintaining your keto diet.

Keep in mind that grocery delivery usually carries a fee and may be more expensive than going to the store, so make sure that you are aware of the cost. If you live in a large city, there may be several different stores that offer grocery delivery that you can check out.

Let others know of your diet

Before going out with friends or going to visit relatives, let them know that you are on the ketogenic diet. Inform them that you don't expect them to prepare any special food for you but that there are many foods that you will not be able to eat. Try to select restaurants that you know have keto-friendly options so that you and your friends can enjoy eating whatever you prefer. And who knows? You may find that others want to join you on the ketogenic diet!

Make friends with others who are on the ketogenic diet

Joining a group of people who are already on the ketogenic diet can be a great way to achieve accountability with people who are working towards the same goals. People who have already been where you are can give you practical advice about how they dealt with the side effects of adjusting to the diet and a state of ketosis, as well as how to handle things like the holidays and those worried emails from your parents about the supposed dangers of going keto. They can also give you pointers about things like saving money on groceries and cooking keto meals separately from what your family normally eats.

While you should avoid preaching to your friends about going keto, some may see how much the diet has benefited you and want to join in. You can hook them up with your buddies who are already on the ketogenic diet and work together as accountability partners.

Exercise regularly

The benefits of exercise are so immense that it is a wonder that doctors don't prescribe it instead of medication. It boosts immunity, improves blood flow and circulation, elevates mood, increases metabolism, burns off the stress hormones that can accumulate after traumatic events or as part of a hectic daily life, burns calories, purges blood sugar, relieves constipation, reduces insulin, the list goes on and on. One reason nutritionists may be against the ketogenic diet is that it doesn't necessarily incorporate exercise.

Going for a brisk walk in the evening or for a morning jog is a great way to get started with exercise. Taking the stairs instead of the elevator and parking further away from the store instead of fighting for a front-row parking spot are easy ways to incorporate exercise into your daily life. You may want to join a gym or buy in-home exercise equipment, but you don't have to. Most people who buy gym membership or exercise equipment never use it unless they were already exercising regularly beforehand.

The best way to make exercise a meaningful and regular part of your life is to make it enjoyable. Put on some music and listen to your favorite songs while you are running on the treadmill. Go for a walk with your family or a friend. You will soon find that you feel so much better, both physically and emotionally, that you will want to continue exercising as much as possible.

Drink lots of water

Because the water-rich foods that you probably once enjoyed, like mangoes and apples, are no longer staples in your diet, you are consuming significantly less water than before. Additionally, when you are first starting out on the ketogenic diet, your kidneys will have to work harder to process all of the fat you are consuming along with the glucose and glycogen stores that your body is burning through. You will have to be intentional about drinking a lot of water. You will probably need to drink one ounce for every pound of body weight. If you are 160 pounds, you will probably need 160 ounces of water per day.

Practice intermittent fasting

Intermittent fasting is the practice of fasting for between 16 and 48 hours at a time for the purpose of gaining health benefits. Intermittent fasting has numerous health benefits. It turns on your body's fat burning processes, improves mental clarity and gets you into a state of ketosis.

You naturally are going into a fasting state at night when you sleep, because you aren't eating. Intermittent fasting extends this state throughout the day. Some experts prescribe fasts as a prelude to beginning the ketogenic diet and others advise fasts as a way to get the most benefits out of it. This is actually much easier than you may think because the ketogenic diet leads to significantly less hunger. When fasting, make sure that you consume plenty of fluids. You may want to supplement with things like coconut oil and butter to help induce ketosis.

Monitor your health

Because the ketogenic diet induces so many chemical changes in your body's metabolism, you need to keep tabs on different markers of health. You can easily buy ketone-testing strips that measure your ketone production through breath, blood, or urine. The ketogenic diet tends to reduce the electrolytes in your body, so you may want to get a tool that measures electrolytes in order to ensure you have an adequate amount. Because the goal of the ketogenic diet is ultimately to suppress the use of glucose for energy by inducing ketosis, you may want to get some tools for testing your blood sugar and insulin levels.

These tools are easily available, as they are frequently used by diabetics as part of their daily regimens.

If implemented correctly, the ketogenic diet can become a lifelong lifestyle of health and wellness that will improve your wellbeing for years to come.

Conclusion

While many people think that weight loss is about just working out, the most important key to shed the pounds is in your own brain. Our brains are made up of our experiences, the things we were taught, the things we've seen, and the biology of our brains provided by ancestors and our parents. Our brains are the most important organ in our body. Without then, we are just bodies. Our bodies are also important, but if we don't take care of our brain, we can't truly take care of the rest.

Weight loss is not a matter of food or exercise; it is a matter of numbers. If you eat too much over a long period of time it will put weight on you. You have to be conscious of what you eat if you have an issue of eating too much, whether it be emotional eating or just not paying attention it is easy to lose sight of what you eat. It is important to be conscious of what you eat every day.

You can enjoy life, eat well, and maintain a good weight that you feel comfortable at and love yourself. It takes a little dynamic thinking, and you can do it.

I believe in you and hope that this book will help you on your quest to find a weight that makes you happy and healthy for life.

Weight loss can be a daunting journey for everyone and it sure seems to require many sacrifices. But it also comes with a promise of a healthy and beautiful body and mind. A weight loss journey is a gradual process and it requires undying patience from you and your loved ones. You may find some days more difficult than others. In those days remember to look back at your achievements as well as your goals. Also realize that weight loss is a personal gain and not something that you do for others. It will only get easier when your body get more used to it. And remember to enjoy the whole process of transformation and be prepared to see yourself in a whole new different light!

Hope this book has managed to unlock the code of weight loss to you in ways that can connect and inspire you. With all the provided information, I wish you success in this self-explorative journey. Good luck!

www.ingramcontent.com/pod-product-compliance
Lightning Source LLC
Chambersburg PA
CBHW062049280526
45788CB00003B/1161